FIGHT!

One Family's Battle
with The Butterfly Disease

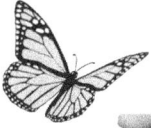

FIGHT!

One Family's Battle
with The Butterfly Disease

VALERIE KALYNKA-BROWN

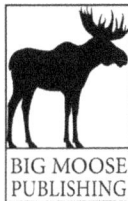

BIG MOOSE
PUBLISHING

Published by:
Big Moose Publishing
234 Pohorecky Street
Saskatoon, SK S7W 0J3
www.bigmoosepublishing.com

ISBN: 978-1-989840-88-7 (sc)
ISBN: 978-1-989840-89-4 (eb)
Big Moose Publishing 08/2025

Dedication

For Marlene

I just finished this book on June 27, 2025, exactly 29 years after we said goodbye. I had made a promise to let your strength be known to the world and I hope this adequately fulfils that promise. I would pick you again to be my sister, and do it all over again in a heartbeat.

Contents

Introduction

The first thing I have to say is that I never thought of myself as a writer, but I have a story that I think needs to be told. My sister, Marlene, was born with a rare skin disease. Marlene's disease is called Recessive Epidermolysis bullosa dystrohica. This type of EB is so rare that only one out of every one million children is born with it. Marlene was definitely one in a million.

This disease is so debilitating that most with it do not make it through childhood. Marlene, however, lived to the age of 37.

Epidermolysis Bullosa (EB) is also called the butterfly disease, because a butterfly cannot be touched without hurting or killing it. A butterfly is beautiful, but very fragile and delicate. This is also the case with those who have this disease. My sister, Marlene, was so fragile and delicate. Her skin, if touched, would blister and tear. If she was touched too harshly, she might not survive her injuries, which could result in death.

In her thirties, Marlene started to write a book while on dialysis in the hospital, twice a week. On her deathbed, I made a promise to her that her book would be published one day. Her book was never finished, but I will continue on with the promise I made to her. Her story will be told.

Before I begin with my version of events, I am including the first chapter of the book Marlene wrote, titled, "Winds of Change". No one can really adequately sum up her view of her life, so I believe her words said in her own way are important to put here.

There is a strange whisper in the wind tonight. As I sit here in complete silence, I hear a soft whisper calling my name. It is also telling me that it's time for a change.

To change in any way, we must first let go of the past. As I sit here and try to make sense of my life, I wonder if there is some purpose to this life that is still unknown to me. Is there something I must do while I am here on this planet? I'm sure we all ask these questions to ourselves at one time or another.

As I look back into my past, I hope to find the answer that will help me understand this unique life of mine. I hope to find some peace in my soul about this life that is a challenge to live. My thoughts immediately drift back to that cold day – January 29, 1959 – the day I was born. Not that I really remember that day, but it is like having a memory of an event because you have been told the story of it over and over again.

No one in my family expected how I would change their lives. My dad was hoping for a boy; that his second child would be a son. Mom was hoping for a quick and easy delivery. My older sister, Darlene, was looking for a playmate. I took everyone by surprise that day.

I was born with a genetic skin disease called Epidermolysis Bullosa (EB). The skin on my entire body, as well as my internal organs, is very sensitive. There is a breakdown of the connective tissue. This means that with only a little pressure or stress on the top, my skin peels off, or I get large water blisters that become open sores. These wounds become easily infected and can be very painful. They can take a week or even months to heal. Some parts of my body are more affected than other parts, due to the re-occurrence of sores in the same area.

My fingers didn't grow past the age of three, and through the years, they have grown together as if encased under a layer of skin. Living with this disease makes me feel like my mind, soul and spirit are trapped in this painful body that makes it very difficult to live my life.

The first few months were tough on me and my parents. I am glad I don't remember much of it. Right after I was born, the doctor accidentally pulled the skin off of my right foot. My mom was horrified to see this and demanded to know how and why the doctor had done this to me, to her baby's foot.

No one quite knew what was wrong with me the first few weeks. I was then sent to the University Hospital in Saskatoon. There, they were able to diagnose my condition, but were really unable to do much for me. They basically told my mom to take me home to die.

They didn't believe I would live very long with this disease. Instead, I surprised everyone with the help and dedication of my parents. Years later, my dad told me that when he looked into my big brown eyes that he knew his little girl would live.

My mom and dad soon realized their brand-new baby girl was not able to breastfeed. I began developing blisters in and around my mouth. They managed to drive to a small town, named Vonda, and ending up knocking on the door of a closed drugstore. The owner of the drugstore opened it up for them, and my mom and dad were able to purchase Olack milk for me. They thanked the store owner and hurried home.

Once my parents were back home, my mom was able to feed me with an eyedropper. My mom said I looked like a little baby bird with my mouth opening waiting to be fed.

The next step was to pad my crib with sponge foam to protect me from hurting myself. Then, my mom had to find a way to stop the blisters from getting larger. She started to break the blisters with a needle. My open sores stuck to my clothes and bedding, and that made them bleed a lot.

One day, my mom remembered that when she was a small child, her father had cut his finger. He pulled out a package of cigarette paper and put the paper over his finger to stop the bleeding and protect the cut. She decided to write the tobacco company and ask if she could get some cigarette paper for her child with a rare skin disease. One day, she had gone to get the mail, and she ended up getting two big rolls of cigarette paper. It was even better, because this paper did not have glue on it like it would if you bought it in the store.

The cigarette paper worked very well. The sores would stay dry, and they could still breathe. When I had a bath, the cigarette paper would eventually come off in the water. Mind you, it would be about a two-hour bath, and then an hour to be re-patched.

I used cigarette paper on my wounds for the rest of my life. All these things my mom did kept me alive. It gave me a chance to fight. I was determined to live no matter what other people thought, and with a lot of care and love, I did live, to the amazement of others.

Those first few years were hard on the family. Mom and Dad didn't go out anywhere for the first two years, because they were afraid to take me anywhere. What if something happened? What if I got hurt or sick? The only time we went anywhere was to the doctor's office. They couldn't help much, but they gave me penicillin to help fight the infections I had.

Our family became separate from most of the outside world. Not many people came to visit, because they didn't know how to react to me. Some people felt sorry for our family, while others thought I was disgusting, and wouldn't look at me, or they would look at me, staring inappropriately. Most of these people saw me as a burden to my family and told my parents to put me in an institution. Sometimes I wondered why they didn't. I know that my mom felt that she would give me the best care. She was right. My mom was very beautiful, but soon she would forget about herself and give up her life in order for me to live.

I learned to talk long before I learned to walk. Mom and Dad both were afraid that I would hurt myself, so they didn't let me out of the crib. I was about the age of two when they had to start letting me try to walk. I did learn how to walk. I would fall, and big blood blisters would form on my hands. Still, even at that early age, I had the determination that nothing would keep me from doing what I wanted to do. Still, learning to walk did leave its mark on me. Every time I fell, the skin between my fingers began to grow together, and this continued to happen through the years, until my fingers were entirely encased in skin.

I eventually lost the use of my fingers, and I had to learn how to do things with my hands. I even had lost all of my fingernails. My toes are the same, but I still tried to continue to run and play like any other child.

Living on the farm at that time did add a few challenges in itself. If I needed a bath, my mom had to draw water from the well, and then warm it up in large pots on the stove. She would let me soak in the tub until the clothes I was wearing would come loose from the sores. This took about an hour.

When all the cigarette paper and clothing came loose, I was able to come out of the tub. I was never able to be towel dried, because it would take more skin off my body and make new sores. When it was time to put new cigarette paper back on all my open sores, it had to be done one piece of paper at a time. Years later, mom would dip the cigarette paper in aloe vera gel, and place it on my blisters. It was like doing papier-mâché.

My mom was kept busy cooking for me, because I was always hungry. This was due to my body needing fuel to heal and fight infections. My mom had a lot on her plate looking after me and my sister, Darlene, and helping my dad on the farm with all the farm animals.

This disease affects all parts of my body. I have experienced all kinds of challenges. I know how it feels to not be able to walk, because the blisters that developed on the bottoms of my feet. Sometimes I would have to sit for days, weeks and months on end. I always tried to walk as soon as I could, so that my bones wouldn't get too weak to carry me.

I have also been blind at times. I would get bad eye colds and infections that would leave my eyelids stuck together and my eyes would hurt too much to open them. I would sit in the dark and listen to the TV all day. I could feed myself with my eyes closed. Most of the time, my eyes would feel better by evening, and I would see again. I would hate to go to sleep for the fear of my eyes being sore in the morning. So, I would stay up late and watch movies on TV. Sometimes this would go on for weeks. Maybe this is why I enjoyed staying up at night. I was never afraid of the dark. Instead, I find the night to be a comfort. It is quiet and peaceful. It is when I can be in touch with myself and the universe.

I also had great trouble eating. My mouth would blister or food would get caught in my mouth and it would be stuck for hours. I sometimes had to wait all day without being able to have one mouthful of water.

I learned early in life to do what I could, when I could, and to be patient, and do other things instead. If I couldn't eat until later, I would play or watch TV, or even have a nap. This made life for the whole family kind of rough and confusing as far as what you did at whatever part of the day or night.

I was said to be a night owl. Like the owl, I always feel best at night. It is the time I feel almost alive. The moon and the stars are entrancing. The night time on the farm can be so quiet and full of secrets. It's almost spooky and kind of haunting. In the night, you can think in peace since most people are asleep. It's the best time to get in touch with your most secret dreams. At night, nothing else is important, not the world or what people think of me. It's the time to look out into the night sky and wonder, "What else is out there in this massive universe?" I feel we must each discover these secrets in our own time and in our own way.

I know I have many secrets to discover for myself about my life and why I am here, living this very challenging life. I have questioned the meaning of my life from a very early age. I hope to find the meaning while writing this book.

But one thing is for certain, no matter how much pain I

have gone through or what has happened, I never knew the meaning of the word defeat. (I hope I never do.)

– Marlene Kalynka

As I mentioned earlier, this is the first chapter of my sister's book. I will continue to put parts of her book in this one as I write. It's the only way anyone can truly understand her pain and determination to live.

Chapter 1

SURVIVING

I often hear people talk about how they want to lose weight or get a nose job. My sister would have jumped into that person's body in a heartbeat. She would have given anything to have healthy, strong skin that wouldn't blister or cause her so much pain and discomfort.

I remember a time when I was trying to ride a two wheel bicycle for the first time. My sister watched me through the living room window as I tried to not fall off. I was finally getting the hang of it when I crashed on the gravel road. I had skinned up my knee pretty badly. My sister, who dealt with this kind of injury over her entire body, was so caring and kind to me. She could have said my whole body is like that 24/7 so get over it, but she didn't.

Looking after Marlene required round the clock – 24 hours a day – care. Our mother would have to tend to Marlene's blisters and wrap them to keep them from getting infected. Living on the farm was challenging for them, since they didn't have running water and there wasn't a bathroom in the house. They did, at least, have power (electricity) in the house.

As Marlene was growing up and having fun playing on the farm, my mom and dad were already planning to move into town. They realized Marlene would not be able to ride the bus to school. Plus, my mom was pregnant with my other sister, Karen, and then a year later, I was born. That was the year that my parents decided to move into town.

They ended up buying a house in Alvena, a small village about 10 miles south of the farm. The house was only one block away from the school. My dad would have to get up very early in the spring time and drive to the farm to go to work. He also had decided to open up a mechanic shop in Alvena. He had gone to GM training school when he was younger, and had become a licensed mechanic. Fixing things came really easy to my father. Years later, when my father was out of town on a hunting trip, the garage burned down. My father never rebuilt it. He said a few people owed him money but only a few came and paid their bills.

I remember the garage fire. I don't know how old I was, but my dad and mom took turns watching the fire out of our kitchen window making sure the fire didn't spread. I was trying to make sense of what was going on. I always remember the one room in that garage. It was filled with every size of tires. Karen and I would go play hide and seek in the room of tires.

Even with us living in Alvena now, Marlene would find it hard to get to school. My mom spent all day looking after Marlene from cooking, cleaning, and bandaging. Plus, she had two younger girls to look after. Marlene getting older didn't make it easier. As Marlene started to age, her disease got worse. I remembered, quite a few times, she couldn't even come out of the bedroom. Her eyes hurt so much from her eye lids sticking together at night. I remember we hung sheets all over the windows to make the house dark, so that she would at least come out of her bedroom.

Every day was a challenge both for Marlene and the family. Some days Marlene could go to school; other days she could not leave her bed. When she did go to school, Marlene wasn't allowed to do everything the other kids did. At recess, Marlene would look out the window of her classroom and watch all the other children playing and running on the playground.

The Alvena School had a desk made that was completely padded so that Marlene could sit in it while in class. It made only a bit of difference, for she was sitting on open sores all day. These wounds would never heal. They would be infected all of her life.

I remember many times if she stepped on a rock or on uneven ground it would cause a huge blood blisters to form on her feet. We had to cut boots and shoes off of her many times.

I was nine years younger than Marlene. I had to be my sister's helper from a very young age. I always look at 9 and 10 year old kids today, and wonder how I did all that. My job was to keep my sister alive by working and cleaning, bathing and bandaging her all the time. Sometimes it felt like my body was there to be her body. If she wanted something done, I often was the one to get up and do it.

I remember Marlene having a bath that took almost 2 hours to soak off all the cigarette paper and a good 30 to 40 minutes to patch and bandage her back up. I would be cutting strips of cigarette paper while she was soaking in the tub. Once she was out of the tub and back on the couch, my job wasn't over. It was an awful job to clean up the tub with all that cigarette paper in the water. It was a job I sure didn't like to do when I was a young girl. I wished I was outside playing and doing kid's stuff like riding my bike.

I never really complained though. I just always did what I

was asked. I was kind of an easy-going little girl. I would watch my poor sister struggle with so many everyday life challenges. Just trying to get dressed or take off her shirt would be a challenge. Every single simple task that most people take for granted as no big deal was always a big deal when it came to Marlene.

Going to the bathroom also was a challenge. Many times, I heard Marlene screaming when she went to the bathroom. Having a bowel movement would cause her so much pain.

Some days her shirt and even the bedding would be stuck to her sores. Imagine not being able to get up because you're stuck, and if you pull your skin comes off or blisters more. It was an insane existence when I think about it now. Also, trying to keep up with the laundry in the house was definitely a challenge. It never ended.

My sister learned from an early age that no one could grab or touch her or she would blister and be in pain. Because of this, she also learned that she could get away with anything. No one could discipline her when she was being bad as a child, or when she didn't want to listen or go to bed. Our father would bundle her up in a big quilt and pretend to throw her down the stairs if she wouldn't listen. She did blame our dad for years to come for being afraid of heights, because of that threat.

Marlene would always try and get her own way. Even

after watching TV, and a program ended, she would cry and scream for mom and dad to put the same show back on. They couldn't, because these were the days before programmed TV and streaming services. Plus, they only had two channels of television to watch.

But, all of these struggles were making her stronger for what lay ahead in her life.

Marlene would spend a lot of her time watching TV and reading books, since most days walking around would only cause more pain. Most of the books and TV shows she found interesting were about animals. Two of her favourite shows were Flicka and Lassie.

She also liked to read about horses. She loved the Black Stallion books written by Walter Farley, and from those stories, she fell in love with the Arabian horse. She even dreamed of owning and riding an Arabian horse one day. This is where the story of passion and courage start to become a reality. This is also where my passion for the Arabian horse comes from.

Here is a snippet of what Marlene wrote about animals, in her own words:

I grew up on the farm until I was 9 years old. I had a great love for animals. They were not just pets to me; they were my friends. I learned quickly that each one of them had their own unique personality.

I remember my first pet cat. She was a grey tabby that we had gotten from my grandfather. I decided to name her Angel. Angel had a quiet nature and liked to sit beside me for hours while I watched TV. She knew not to walk on me and to be careful not to use her claws on me. The cats always jumped over me instead of walking on me. I have always marvelled at the intelligence of our animal friends.

My pets became my best friends for years. I knew they accepted me for me and that they were always loyal.

Something that I really enjoyed was travel. It didn't matter where we went or how far as long as we went for a drive in the car. I would sit happily looking out the window watching for horses. I always found special magic in the beauty of a horse. I also saw grace and strength in them.

My biggest dream at that time was to learn to ride and own my own horse one day. But my parents were too afraid that I would get hurt. So, I kept these dreams a secret, but very much alive, knowing I would fulfil this dream sometime in my future.

Marlene had to learn how to drive a car before she could dream of owning her own horse. Learning how to drive a car was always easier for farm kids. We would learn to drive in the big open fields and never have to worry about hitting anything. As she grew older, Marlene's hands only continued to web together more. You couldn't even tell that at one time she had fingers. This, of course, made learning to drive more of a challenge. She couldn't grip the steering wheel like most people, but she found a way to steer using what she had.

I remember one time the doctors operated on my sister's hands. The doctors had stuck pins through the bones to make her fingers stay straight. When Marlene woke up from the operation, she was horrified, and in so much pain. Eventually, her body started to refuse the pins, and they began coming out of her skin. The pins had to be eventually pulled out putting her in excruciating agony that she shouldn't have had to go through. The whole operation was unsuccessful and her hands continued to close up and web together.

It took my sister seven times to be able to pass her driver's license test. The first six times she went for her driver's test, she failed. The instructors told her that she didn't have any fingers and that she could not grip the wheel properly. But one day my mother made an appointment to take her own driver's test. She told Marlene to go ahead and take her appointment. Marlene did go, and this time – "lucky number seven" – the instructor gave my sister her license to drive. Years later, she would be the one who taught me how to drive. Even the night before I was to take my driver's test, we went out on the highway and she gave me pointers on how to drive. I passed my driver's test on the first try.

Marlene then realized she needed to find a car. She did, and eventually Marlene would move to Saskatoon and finish more of her schooling there. Just the fact that Marlene fought to move out and live independently is a testament to her determination and will. My parents didn't like the idea, but, as always, Marlene got her way. She then worked on fulfilling her dream to ride a horse, and maybe even own one.

Finding a car for Marlene to drive was much easier than finding a horse for her to ride. Most places to go ride horses or take riding lessons were way out of town. Marlene eventually was able to find a nice man named Ken who owned Appaloosa horses. He said he could pick her up in town and drop her off after her lesson. So, Marlene would take a taxi or the bunny bus (for disabled people) and met Ken at the end of the city. He would pick her up and take her to his place so that she could ride.

Marlene would stand on a chair, and with the help of Ken, she would get up in the saddle. Then, he would just walk the horse around and around the ring until the lesson was over. Marlene loved every minute of this. She would feel so normal to be able to ride a horse. She was on cloud nine.

Marlene started looking for other places to ride. She found a therapeutic riding place that also would let her get on a horse. There, she was able to ride a white Arabian gelding named Rip. Her dreams of Arabian horses were starting to come true.

The hunt was on to find her the perfect Arabian horse she could ride and own. I was in Alvena and going to school during the week, and then I would go to Saskatoon on the weekends and for the summer to help Marlene, when she wouldn't have home care.

We kept a close eye on the local newspapers looking for ads of horses for sale. If Marlene thought the horse was good, we would go out and see it. We started a diary that I still have to this day. I would write on one page about the horse and if I thought it would be a good fit. And she would write on the opposite page about the horse. I was always the first to ride the horse. I would help make the decision whether Marlene should get on and ride or not. This was a very important decision, because if she got hurt by falling off the horse, she probably would not have lived through her injuries.

A lot of people were really helpful with letting Marlene take a horse for two weeks to try It out. Most of those horses would have been fine for me, but they were not quite gentle enough for Marlene.

We toured all over Saskatchewan and even Alberta trying to find the perfect horse. I remember one well broke quarter horse gelding. I think he was a buckskin. He would move and turn on a dime for me, but when my sister got on, he knew right away that she didn't have much strength to control him. Marlene was 5'7" and weighed only 80 lbs. She just wasn't strong enough to handle him.

I remember another horse named Kelly. She had some Arabian blood in her. Maybe she was even a purebred. The owner told me I could go ride her out in the big field. I took her for a good run, but then, of course, she took off real fast back to the yard. I was riding fine until she saw a spot in the tree to the opening of the yard, which took me by surprise. I ended up on the ground, and I was knocked out for a few seconds. Marlene did not get on this horse. But the owner did say he used to race this mare through the fields with his buddies on horseback.

Sometimes these horses were just not safe enough for me to ride either. I also remember a younger mare that I rode. She was doing good and then just decided to buck on the spot. I wasn't sure what to do, so I just jumped off. Marlene would always laugh when I hit the ground coming off the horse. I never liked that. I didn't think it was very funny. Luckily, I never got hurt.

Marlene would wear winter mitts, ski pants and a helmet when she rode. She still would get blisters from the friction of the horse while riding. She would even wear the ski pants when she rode in the hot summer months, but she was so happy to be able to ride a horse and feel normal, it was worth going through the heat and pain to her.

Driving home from Saskatoon one day, Marlene finally had the courage to tell our dad that she was looking to buy a horse. She did not know how Dad would react to this, but she knew she had to tell him. The conversation started off a bit rocky, but Marlene was determined to get a horse. Finally, my dad said, "Look, there are two horses in the field over there. We can pull in and see if they are for sale. Immediately, I started to cry, thinking this would really be happening. But Marlene told our dad she was looking for something specific and safe to ride. She wasn't going to settle for just anything.

CHAPTER 2

OUR MOM

It takes a special kind of person to be an EB mom. My mom grew up in Cudworth, Saskatchewan. Her mom and dad were both Ukrainian. They had seven kids, of which my mom was the second oldest. She lived a hard life on the farm doing chores, going to school and helping her mother with her younger brothers and sisters.

She would tell me stories of how all her brothers and sisters would sleep in one bedroom. I remember her telling me a story of how her younger sister had burnt her arm on the woodstove. The burn was pretty bad. My mother would soak off the bandages while her sister was sleeping and my mother would re-bandage it. She said the burn was severe and got infected. Little did my mother know or understand at the time what she would be in for in her life with regards to blisters and bandaging. My sister's body had about 50% of it raw with blisters. In fact, a lot of people did think my sister was burnt in a fire, but she was born this way.

The care and dedication my mom gave my sister was truly remarkable. My mother who was an absolutely beautiful woman and who got married at the age of 21, had no idea what her life was going to become. I remember so many times coming home for lunch from school to find my poor mom fast asleep on the couch, exhausted from looking after Marlene all night. I would quietly find myself something to eat and head back to school. We never really had breakfast or suppers. My mom just physically did not have the time to do that. We just ate when we could around Marlene's schedule.

My mom knew quite quickly how to look after Marlene. Most of the doctors and nurses didn't understand, and maybe didn't want to. I remember a doctor giving my sister one tiny tube of antibiotic cream and my sister got mad. This wouldn't even cover one spot on her back, let alone her whole body. My mother and sister fought with the doctors and nurses constantly, because they just didn't comprehend the amount of care she needed.

My mom didn't have time to look after herself either. She never learned to drive a car and never got her license. She had only completed her grade 8 education. Back in those days you had to stay home and help around the house doing the cooking, cleaning and chores. And then with Marlene, and 3 other children to care for, her whole life revolved around her children, particularly Marlene.

My mother's life was definitely a challenge, but she just kept doing the best she could with what she had.

EB is a hereditary disease. My mom did have two miscarriages after Marlene was born. There definitely could have been more of her children with this disease. I do thank my lucky stars that I wasn't born with EB. I have always felt a bit guilty, because I was born healthy and had beautiful skin. I think my sister believed if she had been healthy, she would have been like me. We did share many interests, including the love of animals and living the farm life.

My mom never really had any help with Marlene other than the little we tried to give her. But we were just kids ourselves. There weren't any supports or programs available like we have today. My mother did the best she could for our family, even if she fell behind in so many other ways.

My mom was amazing, and she was my best friend. When she finally went into a nursing home after my dad passed, I would call her every day. I would say, "What are you doing?" and she would say, "Do....ing?" and then she'd say,

"Sitting by the phone waiting for you to call." I wouldn't trade my mother for any other mother in the world. I think about her every day and miss her so much.

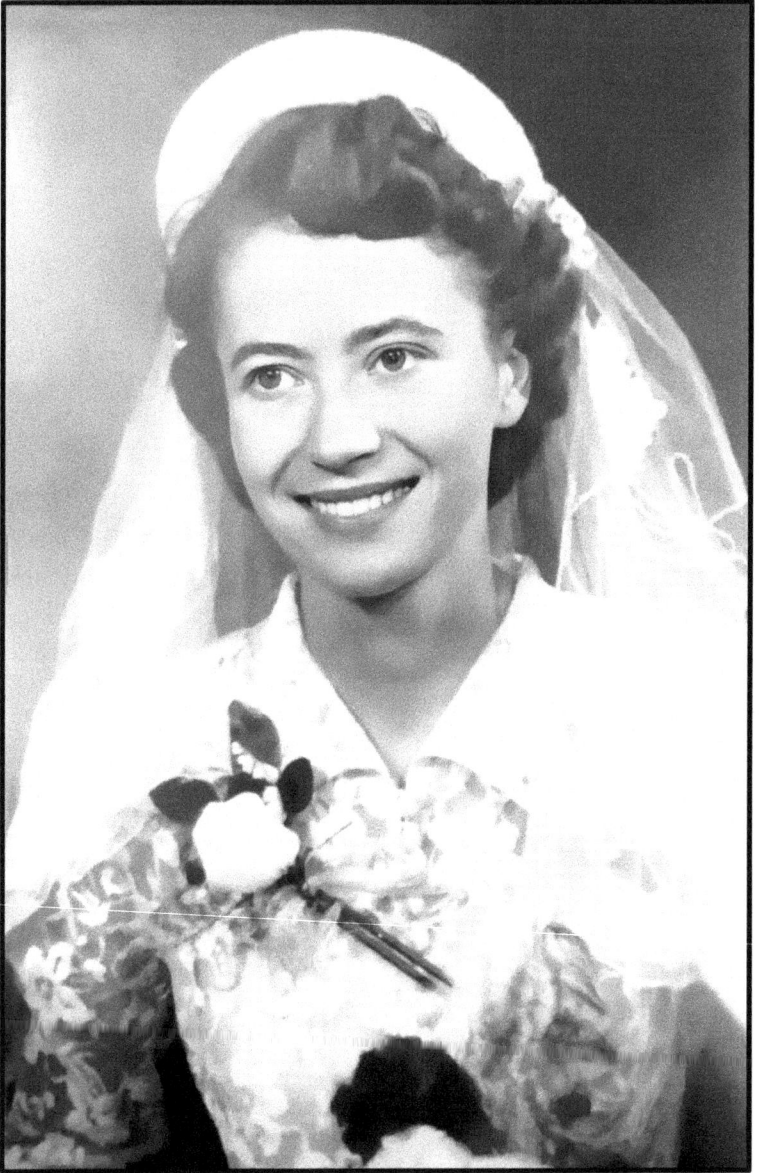

Our mom on her wedding day

CHAPTER 3

ABOUT ME

I was the youngest in our family and was nine years younger than Marlene. When I was reading Marlene's writings after she passed, I found this: "I looked down in the crib at Valerie and saw in her eyes that she and I would have a special relationship." She also wrote, "Thank God for Valerie."

Marlene and I seemed to have the same love and interests, like a love for animals, especially horses. I spent a lot of time as a child chasing birds and cats and dogs in our small town. By the time I was about nine years old, I started to become my sister's helper. Marlene was eighteen. Whatever my sister needed or wanted, I was the kid who would go and do it for her.

Back then, we never had a remote to change the TV channels. I was the one to get off my chair and always change the TV channel for her. I also learned at a really young age how to cook for and bandage my sister. Cooking was tough. If I cooked scrambled eggs too long, the eggs would become too hard and would cause my sister's mouth to form water blisters in it. Then, she would have to poke them with a needle. So many times, I would have to remake the food I had cooked for her.

I totally became her hands and feet. It was like my body became her body. I remember not being able to sit on the couch long before she would have me up doing something for her that she couldn't do.

Giving my sister a bath could take up to 4 hours from start to finish. Being a young kid, I didn't get a chance to do some of the things I wanted to do. I really didn't mind helping my sister, but as I was getting older and becoming a teenager, I started to want to be my own person. I wanted to go to school dances, and I wanted to hang out with friends. It was really hard to do because she wanted to come with me, or she didn't want me to go. I remember having to start a fight just so I could go do the things I wanted to do.

My sister was not used to someone telling her no. A few times, she would get so mad at me for not doing what she wanted me to do, that she would either wreck my things or she would throw my things away. The older I became, the more I realized that I didn't really know who I was. Did I like horses and animals because she did? Did I really like the TV shows or were they just ones she liked? Did I even know what was my favourite colour? I had been so busy looking after everything she liked and needed that I was lost.

Once Marlene moved to the city, I would only go on the weekends to look after her. My mom would find me a ride Friday after school. I would stay at Marlene's apartment and cook and clean and look after her cat…every weekend. I would call a taxi if we were going somewhere for a doctor's appointment. I would even have to call 911.

My parents would come on Sunday to pick me up. Marlene would again have my mom so busy to get her ready for the week on her own. She did have some home care come in during the week, but every Sunday night we wouldn't get back home until midnight. Then, I had to somehow get up early the next morning to go to school.

I never really liked school, but most of the time I was just too tired to care about it. With not eating the best and not getting enough sleep, school was just a place I had to go. Most kids and people that lived in our small town really didn't understand what was going on in our household. Our family was just struggling to help my sister live.

My sister would eat so slowly. It would take her all night to eat and then she would be hungry for more. My mother would be up all night looking after Marlene. Our whole household was dysfunctional. We would be teased at school, because people didn't understand what was really going on. People saw that my sister looks different, but had no clue that her whole body was covered in infected open sores. I wouldn't wish this disease on even my worst enemies.

I took on the role of my sister's helper whether I wanted to or not, but I don't regret giving up my childhood to help her, and I would do it all over again.

CHAPTER 4

OUR DAD

My father was born on a farm just northwest of Alvena, Saskatchewan. He was the mayor of Alvena for 25 years. He had attended GM training school in Saskatoon and became a mechanic. Mechanics came easy to him. He loved to help people and never charged much money to fix things for them.

I remember a story my dad once told me. He had been working in the field with his family. He was pitching wheat into the thrashing machine with a pitchfork. He was probably in his early 20s or maybe younger. When he went to throw the pitchfork full of wheat at the thrash machine, it somehow hit the belt and the handle of the pitchfork came flying back at him. The handle hit him hard in the chest, knocking him to the ground. Everyone ran to him and found that he wasn't breathing. His heart had stopped. My dad told me when this happened that he had felt so peaceful. He was going somewhere; he was following a light. He said it was like nothing he had felt before, and he didn't want to go back. But somehow, he did come back. His heart started to beat again and he was breathing. His mother thought for sure he was dead.

My father came back to life, thankfully, or I would not be here today. He said he always felt like he came back to be able to help other people. There wasn't a farm around Alvena that my dad hadn't been to help fix something whether it be a car, a truck, or farm machinery. Our phone at home rang all the time for someone wanting my dad to go and fix something. My dad was always working and smiling. We never saw him much since he would be gone to the farm early in the morning, and come home late at night. He worked very hard to support his family.

I had moved to Ontario in 1992. I was the daughter that was supposed to take over the family farm, but somehow I ended up moving to Ontario. I still often wonder how I ended up here. I never thought I would leave Saskatchewan. My mother always told me that Saskatchewan was the safest place to live.

I watched my father turn into an old man in the three years after my sister had passed away. He always felt so guilty bringing a child into this world that had to suffer so much in pain. My sister had passed away in 1996. In 1999, my father decided to follow her into the heavens above.

My father was a very talented man. He played in a band called The Happy Ramblers. He had taught himself to play the guitar, drums, and banjo. He also could sing.

My Dad lost his father when he was five years old. He was a great dad, even though he ended up growing up without a father himself. His father, my grandfather, was crossing the river going to or from Rosthern and the horse and wagon broke through the ice. He died due to falling in the freezing cold water. This was in 1922. Then my dad's youngest brother, Nick, who was just a baby when his father had died, was also taken away at 18 years old from a ruptured appendix. Nick was 5 years younger than my dad and loved horses. My dad said he could walk in any field and catch any horse, while the horse would just run away from him. Horses were in Nick's blood just like they are in mine and Marlene's.

One night, my dad was woken up by his mom saying Nick was really sick. She told him to go get the horses ready to take him to town. My dad hitched up the horses and buggy in the middle of a cold, January night and got Nick to the train station in Alvena to get him to the doctor in Saskatoon.

Nick arrived at the hospital, but there was a young doctor working. He told my dad and his mother to donate their blood to Nick, because his appendix had burst. It was too late. Nick never made it, and he died on January 16, 1939.

I always found it kind of odd and strange, don't know what to call it, but I was born with horses in my blood, too, on January 16th.

***

After my father passed, Alvena would have a new mayor. This new mayor approached our family and told us he was going to make a park in Alvena. He also wanted to name the park after Marlene. The new park had opened and it was even on the local news. On TV, people from our small town finally were able to see how my sister had been covered in blisters all her life and how much pain she had been in. A friend of my dad's said that he had no idea she was covered in sores and blisters.

I will always be grateful for my dad. I remember I was begging him to buy me my first horse, Gypsy. He had said that we had nowhere to keep a horse. The farm had no well on it and no corrals. He told me to go ask a cousin who was also the principal of our school if I could keep my horse on his farm. So I did. I walked up to my cousin at school and asked if I could keep a horse at his place and he said yes. I was so excited and couldn't wait to go home from school to tell my dad.

My dad was shocked that I asked him. Then, the next day I asked my dad if he would buy me the horse. My dad opened his wallet and started handing me fifty dollar bills to pay for the horse. I started to cry. My first horse was delivered the next day.

I am thankful to my dad and cousin Ernie for getting me started on my journey that turned out to be a life long passion with horses. I will always have a horse, especially an Arabian horse.

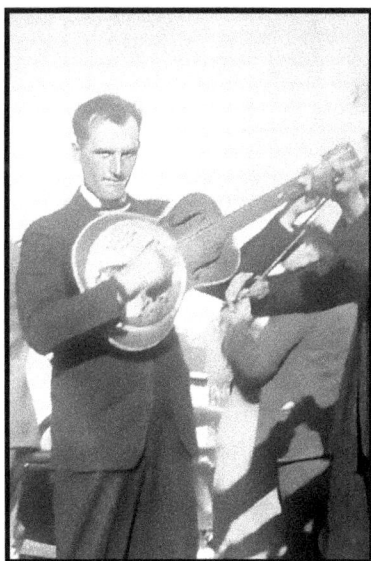

Our dad playing with his band

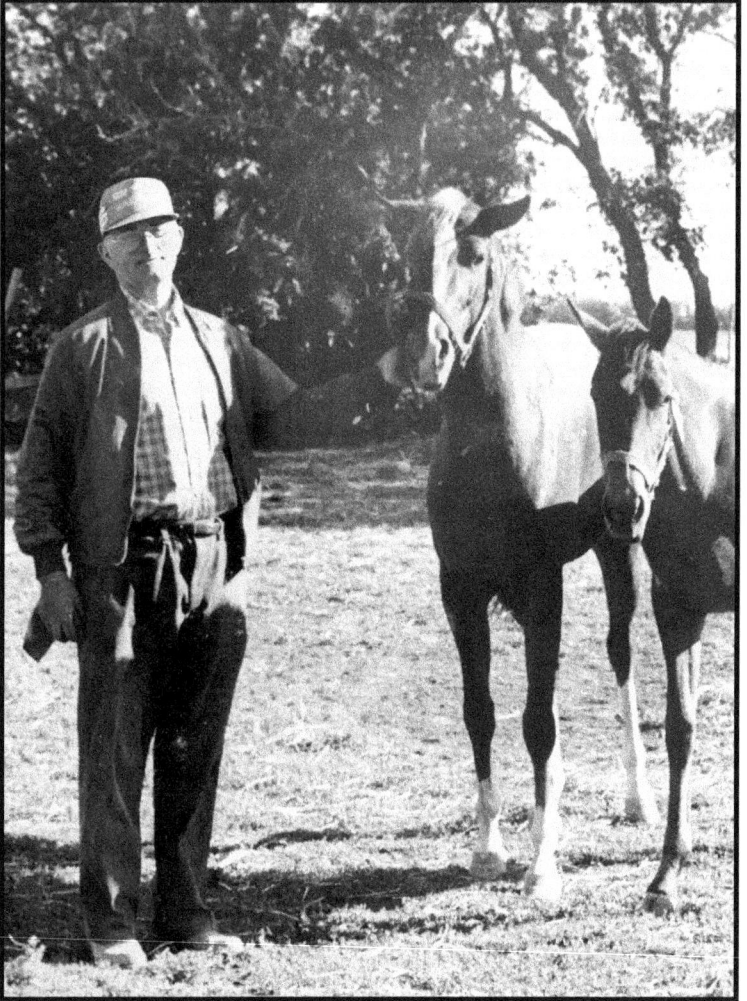

Dad with horses

Chapter 5

HORSES, HORSES, HORSES

Finally, after searching for the perfect horse for Marlene to ride, we found a little Arabian mare that was trained really well, but had just been a brood mare for quite a few years. The mare was a liver chestnut with a blonde mane and tail, and only 13 hands high. She was bred and was due to foal the following spring. Her name was Basheerah.

When we went to go pick up this mare, my sister's friend's husband drove his truck and trailer to get it. It was early morning and still dark out. The truck and trailer were running outside the front of his house. When we walked outside to leave, the truck had rolled down the hill a bit, and had hit a tree. Luckily, the truck wasn't damaged. Maybe the grill was a little banged up, but nothing major, thank goodness.

We brought the little mare home. They were letting my sister try her out for two weeks. I could ride her no problem and get her to jog really slowly. My sister could ride her, but she found trotting to be hard and it was hurting her body. I told Marlene to just stand up a bit in the stirrups, because it seemed too slow the horse down.It worked the mare didnt have to be sent back to the owner.Marlene then purchased this little mare.

Basheerah delivered her foal on April 20th. I remember the date because Marlene and I would go out to the barn every night and wait to see foal being born. Early in the morning on April 20th, my sister and I got to see a beautiful liver chestnut filly be born. I even remember the song playing on the radio that morning. It was Juice Newton's "Just Call Me Angel" and the lyrics go "just call me Angel of the morning".

Everything was going well with Basheerah, but once her foal was weaned, she seemed to have gotten a mind of her own. She was still really good for my sister to ride though.

She then started to test me. I remember getting on her bareback in a big indoor arena and she decided to run off with me. There were some of fairly high jumps in the arena. Of course, she ran straight to them and stopped dead, which I then somehow ended up standing on my two feet right behind her. I am not even sure how that happened.

One day, I was riding Basheerah in the arena and a couple of ladies walked in. The one lady said, "Oh my goodness, that horse is BonBon". All I could think was that the horse was named Basheerah. The lady then told us she was a sister of the lady who sold us the horse. She proceeded to tell us that this little mare used to try to kill her. She said she would run through the trees, water, and roads to try to get her off her back. Things were starting to make sense of how this little horse would treat certain people. I then knew I was her next victim.

Basheerah was a pure bred registered Arabian and knew exactly what her rider could handle. I could ride her just fine, and then just out of the blue, she would take off with me at a full gallop. Finally, one day I was tired of her doing this, so I reached down and grabbed her bit with my hand and pulled her sharply around. That was the end of her running away with me. Interestingly, she never tried any of this with Marlene. She behaved like a really good little horse with her. Marlene could walk, trot and gallop in the indoor arena. She could go with me and another horse on a trail ride, and Marlene even rode her in an Arabian horse show.

Marlene had no fingers to be able to grip the reins. So, her reins had been altered so that she could have loops attached, and she put her hands through the loops. Luckily Marlene never really got hurt riding, but one fall would have more than likely killed her. She most likely would not have survived the injuries. Still, she ended up having and riding this mare for over 10 years. Over that time, my love for the Arabian horses grew too. I ended up owning a part bred Arabian mare named Gypsy, and then a pure bred mare named Cindy.

I even ended up going to Oklahoma to become a farrier. A farrier is someone who shoes horses. This is something my sister never knew I did, but she would have loved it. Horses were in our blood. Both my mom and dad told me that my grandfathers on each side also loved horses. My dad's father had a pair of white horses that he only harnessed to take people to funerals and weddings. My mom's father also loved horses, so I definitely see where this passion comes from.

To this day, I still have Arabian horses. After I lost my horse named Valdor, an Arabian I had for 34 years from birth, I knew in my heart that I needed another Arabian horse to have in my life. I looked at a few. I liked them all, but I looked up to the sky and said, "Marlene give me a sign of which horse I am supposed to buy". Then, a lady whose two horses I had looked at that were for sale, sent me a video of a couple month old colts which had caught my eye when I had visited her earlier. She said in the video that one of the colt's names was Farley. I knew right then and there what to do. Walter Farley had written the Black Stallion books which made my sister fall in love with the Arabian breed. I bought him, and I love him. I knew my sister had sent me the sign.

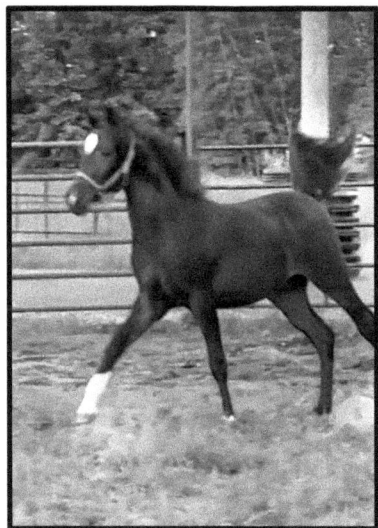

Farley

Another sign from my sister came when I was deciding whether or not to write this book. I looked up in the heavens above again and said, "Let me know if I am supposed to write this book." One morning, in 2024, I was having coffee and was on Facebook. I was reading about a lady asking about an Arabian stallion her father used to own. She wanted to know if anyone knew more info about her dad's stallion. I started to read the comments. I couldn't believe my eyes. She said that her dad's stallion had a sister named Basheerah.

Such a small world! The lady who made the post and I hit it off instantly. We texted and found out her Arabian stallion also knew how to read people. He was so good with her as a child and could dislike strangers. I knew then this book had to be written.

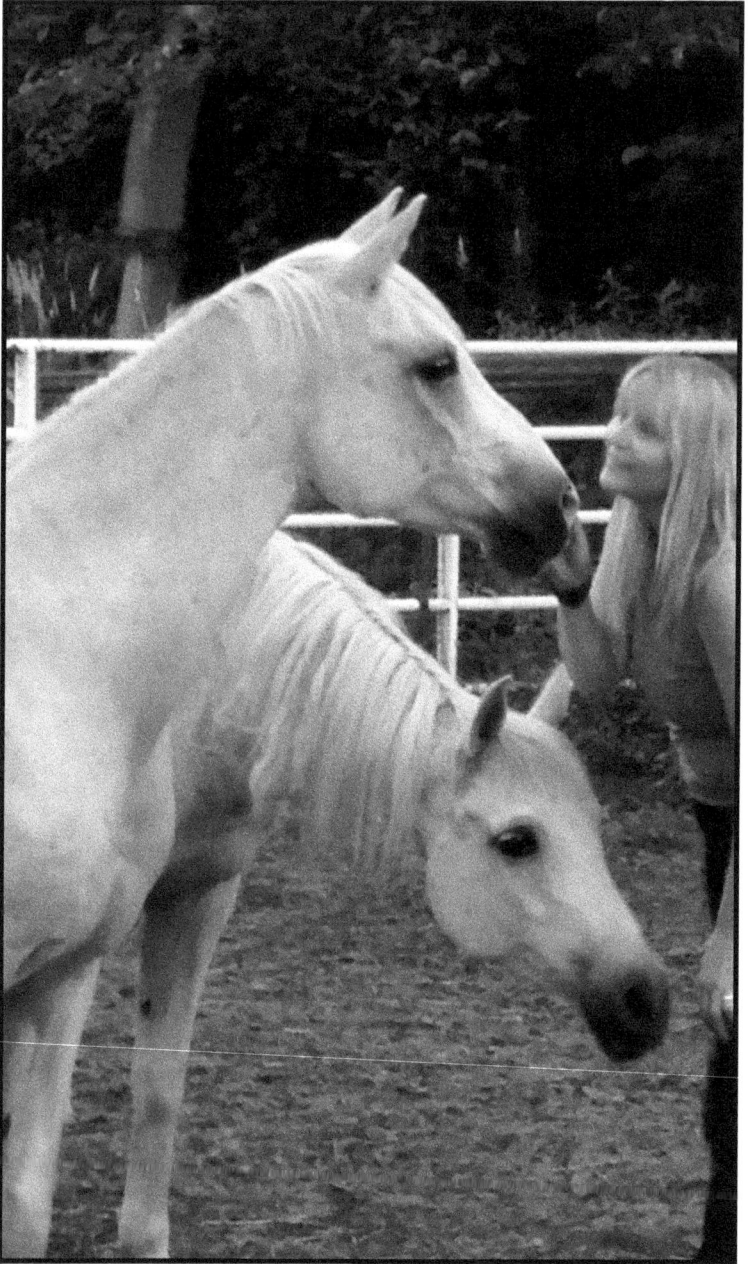

Me (Valerie) with Valdor and his full sister, Lacey

Chapter 6

CHANGES COMING

As I got older, I started to pull away from my sister. I was trying to figure out who I was and what I wanted out of life. My sister also was starting to change direction. She had more of her own friends and was really liking music. She went to see many bands and artists live. She even decided to start taking drum lessons. She would use a band on her wrist and put the drumsticks underneath them to hold them in place. She, again, was proving to the world that being physically challenged was not going to stop her from what she wanted to do.

I was still into horses and had a boyfriend. We were starting to breed Arabians and Appaloosas. We had spent many days in the field with my dad making hay to feed these horses.

Marlene and I were fighting more, because she still wanted my help, and tried to demand it. I was on a path to find my own identity. We even got into a big fight the week I was to graduate from grade 12. She also picked a fight with my boyfriend at the time and said she wasn't going to my graduation if he was going. Then my other two sisters took her side, also. As it worked out, my whole family and boyfriend were at my graduation, but most of them weren't speaking to me.

I learned so much from my sister Marlene, but she could be very demanding to get her way. Her passion for horses was getting put on the back burner and music was becoming her priority. She had really started to meet friends. She had met one friend at a concert and, to this day, I still talk to him about the friendship they had. He even wrote a song about my sister. (Note: Marlene legally changed her name to Oceania later in life. That is why this song is titled Oceania.)

OCEANIA

I've never met someone
I'll never meet anyone
Quite like you again
Sitting together as
Concert lights go down
In an instant, a bond
Between strangers begins
Everlasting friendship
We were riding the wind
Oceania

We never really know
How much time
We have on this
Rock called Earth
All I know is
I wanna spend as much time
As I possibly can with you
Never asking anything
From each other,
We wanted to stand together
As kindred souls
Oceania

Life's long drives
back and forth
We were listening to that
Thing called rock 'n' roll, so indeed
We turned the volume up
Not a single care
We were singing like two graceful birds
Never noticed how far
For we were counting above
Those beautiful stars
Oceania

I wasn't there when you
Decided to close your whirlwind eyes
Memories I carry
Never to let go
I envision places you've stood
Each time I still breakdown
My friend, I can still feel you around me
Though we never said it
I truly loved you
I hope you found peace
Your Shangri-La with no pain
To see each other once again
We will blare that music
Up ever loud just once again
For being with you
A second time around will be such a charm

Certain days out of the blue
I just break down like a knight
Laying upon their sword
After all this time
I just end up missing you more and more
So I've written these words down for you
My friend always
Oceania

Rene CC
March 17, 2025

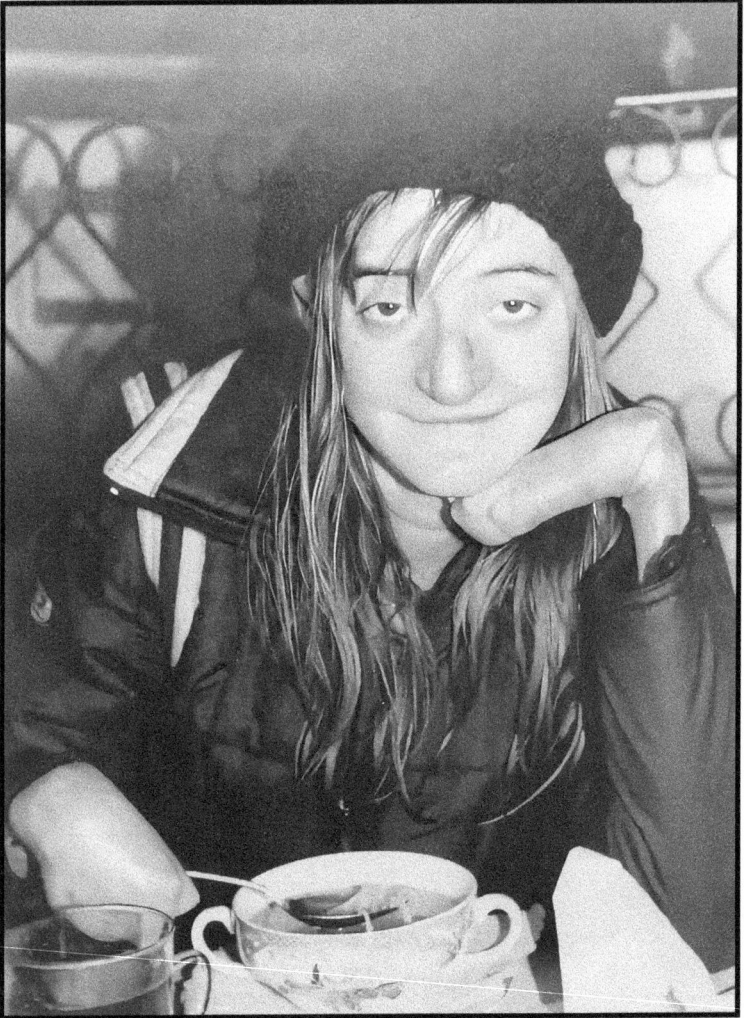

Marlene

Chapter 7

MOVING

Marlene finally decided to sell her horses and move to Toronto. She wanted to go to music school. Again, she was defying the odds of what anyone thought she was capable of. My boyfriend at the time that was raising horses and farming with and I had mutually decided to part ways also. I was also starting to change my life. I was selling a few horses, and then somehow I ended up moving to Ontario not too long after my sister did.

I moved to London, Ontario. Marlene had bought herself a car in Toronto and decided to drive out to London to visit me, not long after I moved there. She drove by herself on the 401 highway, for two hours, and made it to the mall I was working in. She stayed a couple of days. I was able to take her to a stable where my horse, Valdor, was boarded at. Valdor was my pure bred Arabian gelding who I had shipped from Saskatoon. Marlene was quite impressed with Valdor. She thought he was a beautiful horse.

When it was time for Marlene to head back to Toronto, she felt too tired and didn't think she could make the drive back by herself. So then, I had to drive her back two hours to Toronto. I was nervous, because I had never driven on such a big highway with so many cars. But she just pushed me to do things that I may or may not have wanted to do. This was what my childhood was like. If she told me to climb the tallest tree and jump, she could make me do it.

Our relationship had changed as I started to grow up. I was finally standing up for myself and it was not easy. I wanted to help her, and felt guilty that I also wanted to find myself. Marlene and I were really close and shared a special bond, but we also had moved in different directions.

When Marlene had moved to Toronto, she also legally changed her name to Oceania. Boy, did she get mad at us if we still called her Marlene. She probably is mad in heaven right now that I am using Marlene more in this book than Oceania, but I think she will forgive me.

When Marlene had moved to Toronto, I remember going to her place to see her. I hadn't seen her for a couple of months and was excited to visit with her. She was on the phone. It was about 9:00 pm and she was talking to a guy she liked. I asked her where I could sleep, since I had to get up at 4:00 am to catch a flight back home to Saskatoon. She never got off the phone. I fell asleep on the corner of the couch. Finally, when it was 4:00 am, she said to wake up and to make her bed. I quickly made her bed, called a taxi, and ran out the door. I remember feeling hurt that she never got off the phone to talk to me.

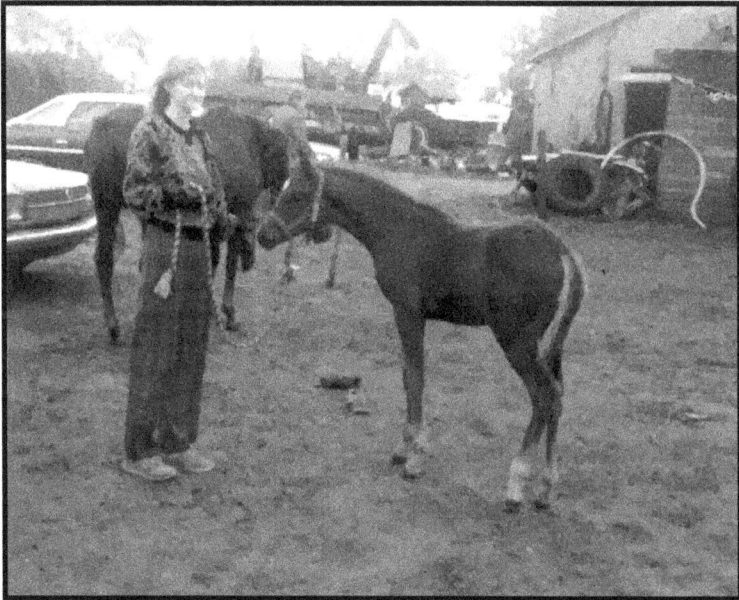

Marlene with colt that she named Never Surrender after one of her favourite sayings and songs

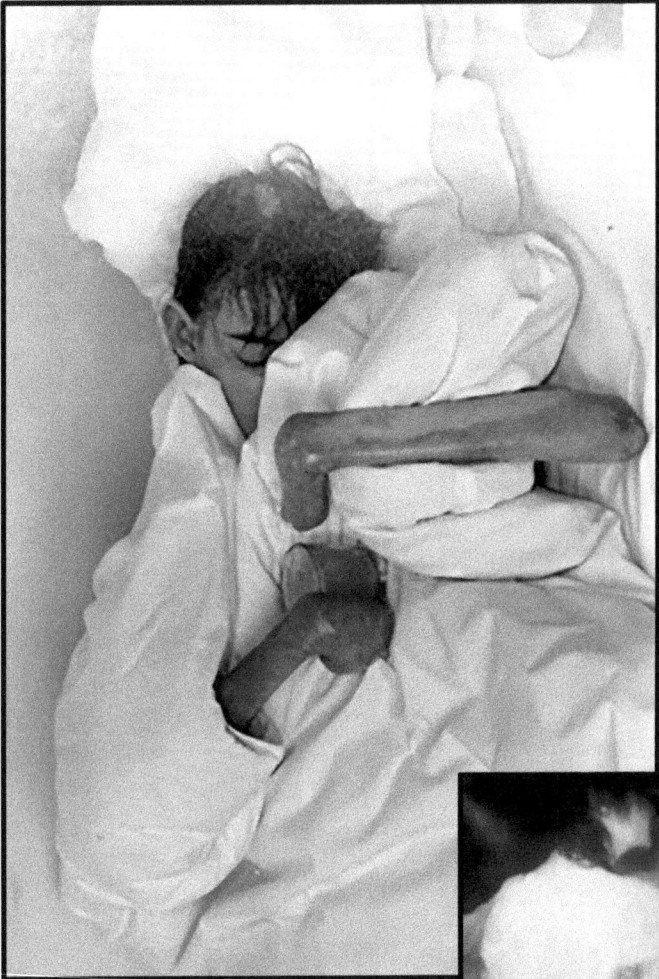

Marlene taking a nap

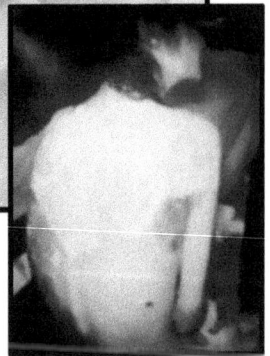

Marlene's back covered in cigarette paper to cover her open sores

Chapter 8

THE HARD PARTS

I thought I was totally done writing this book when I talked to a soul sister from another mother. She said one thing we all have in common is that we are human. I was telling her of the hard parts of my life and about my sister and how hard she could be on me. She told me to add this chapter in my book. I didn't want to write anything bad about my sister, because she was such an inspiration and her determination to live and do was beyond what I will ever see in my life. She was incredibly resilient, but she did have a mean side to her. If she wanted something, she was determined to get it, no matter who got in the way.

Since I was nine years younger than Marlene, I really was just a kid that had to take a lot of responsibility on at an early age. I was a very happy-go-lucky kid, so I just did what I was told. I do look at 9 to 12 year old kids today and think of the stuff I did at their age. They would never be able to do what I did.

One summer, however, my sister went away to Germany for a treatment of her disease. It was the first time I ever had a summer to myself. I woke up early and would go to the farm with my dad. I saddled up and rode my Arabian mare named Cindy without worrying about what Marlene needed. I really enjoyed not having to look after my sister, and loved not having to do what she wanted me to do.

When she came home after two months, I no longer wanted to be at her beck and call. I wanted to do other things. I wanted to go to a school dance without her, because she would make me dance with her, and I would get teased by the other school kids. Back then, kids teased us about anything and everything, and were ruthless. I would start a fight with her just so that I could go without her. Of course, she would get mad and get into stuff and she would wreck my artwork and flush my earrings down the toilet. So, as inspirational as she was, she was not a saint.

I remember one time she was chasing me around the house and told me to get outside. I told my dad to make her stop or I was going to throw something at her and hurt her. My dad said, "Don't do it. There is nothing to throw at and it will hurt her."

One day she just kept pushing me and pushing me. I finally stuck my hand in a nearby plant, grabbed a handful of dirt, and threw it in her face. She stopped dead in her tracks and just stared at me. I felt awful the minute I did it, but I just couldn't and wouldn't be controlled in the same way anymore. I was starting to stand up for myself and figure out who I was. I think a few days later, she told me it really shocked her, that I would throw dirt in her face. She said no one had ever stood up to her before and done something like that. I was thankful that I only shocked her, and that I did not hurt her. The only thing I hurt was her pride.

I also remember my 13th birthday. I was sitting in the living room and was excited. I was turning into a teenager. Marlene asked me to make cookies for her, and I said I would, even though no one was making me a cake or cookies for my birthday. It was around supper time and my dad had come home from the farm. He sat at the table eating when I went over to sit by him and tell him excitedly that it was my birthday. My dad grumbled something and kind of snapped at me and said it's not your birthday. I felt hurt and ran off to my bedroom. The next thing I know Marlene was running after me screaming and yelling at me to make her cookies. She screamed and kicked my door until it was two or three in the morning until my dad finally got up and yelled at her to go to bed. Other kids turning 13 had birthday cakes and gifts. All I got was no sleep.

Growing up in our house, it seemed we always were short one bedroom. This meant that when I had outgrown my crib, from then on, I never had anywhere to sleep. I didn't have my own bedroom until I was probably 13 years old. I slept on the couch, the floor, and even in the closet. I remember being tired all the time. When I got up to go to school, I would have a coffee and some bread and butter, and then would run down the back alley to go to school.

Looking back, it's no wonder I hated school and didn't do well. I was exhausted and had no nutrition in me. After school, my sister and I would go to the co-op and buy pop, chocolate or chips for our supper. Our family was dysfunctional with Marlene's conditions and with her running the household. My poor mom was also exhausted trying to keep up with the demands of Marlene's condition.

There was one summer when I went with Marlene to West Germany for her treatments. At the time, I was 14 years old. I was supposed to be her helper way across the ocean. Once we arrived in Frankfurt, Germany, we took a taxi to a small town where the clinic was located. We got Marlene settled in. Darlene had also come and was going to be leaving only after a week or so. I ended up staying there for a month.

I remember seeing so many kids and adults with skin diseases at the treatment centre. I remember this cute little girl in ponytails who had something called fish skin disease. It was like her body was covered in fish scales, but she was such a cute bright-eyed girl. Others that had EB were wheelchair bound. Some had feeding tubes. Some had no hair on their heads or bald spots, and most of them didn't have any teeth. I do have to say some of them were hard for me to look at.

My sister's condition never bothered me, because I was used to seeing her like that. While Marlene was doing her treatments, which included a very strict diet, homemade everything, her sores started to heal up. She also had certain kinds of creams to apply to her sores. She was starting to feel better and wanted to go out a bit to see the sites.

I remember us finding a pub opened in one of the malls. There was a band and what she thought was a cute lead singer. So, of course, we went in. I at 14 had to pretend I was 18, which wasn't hard because I looked about 18 years old. The pub was filled with a bunch of American soldiers that kept coming by and hitting on me. I was so uncomfortable and completely terrified.

One afternoon, after leaving the pub, the singer of the band was by the sidewalk we were standing on, and about to leave, when my sister decided to jump in the front seat of his friend's Volkswagen Beetle. There I was, standing in the middle of the road, wondering what to do. The car was now full of guys I didn't know and my sister. I was going to be left behind by myself or I had to get into the backseat and sit on some guy's lap I didn't know. I also couldn't let my sister go off by herself. She could get hurt. She many times would get locked in the bathroom and not be able to undo a lock, because it would blister her hands. So, I jumped in the car.

The next thing I realised was that all these guys and the driver were drunk or high on drugs. We were heading onto the Autobahn where cars drive as fast as they can go. The driver was definitely driving his Volkswagen bug as fast as it could go. I was a bit scared, but we did live through it, thank God.

***

My sister was hard on me, but she helped me to become who I am today. I was a very responsible child and still am to this day. She wasn't perfect, but really want people to know how inspirational she was and about how she did things people didn't think she could do because of her condition.

I could also have been born with this disease. Some family have more than one child needing this kind of care from this disease. Some people only get this disease in their hands and feet. Others have blisters, but not as severe as my sister had. My sister had blisters on her entire body inside and out. What's interesting is that horses can get EB too, but are euthanized at birth.

I always thought I would have children, but that just wasn't in the cards. I could've also had a child with EB, because it is hereditary. I think maybe I didn't have children because I had already been a kid with a mother's responsibility. Not having kids has given me the freedom to do what I want as an adult, and enjoy life differently. I am grateful to have had Marlene in my life, and if I had the chance to do it all over again, I would have to say, "You betcha!"

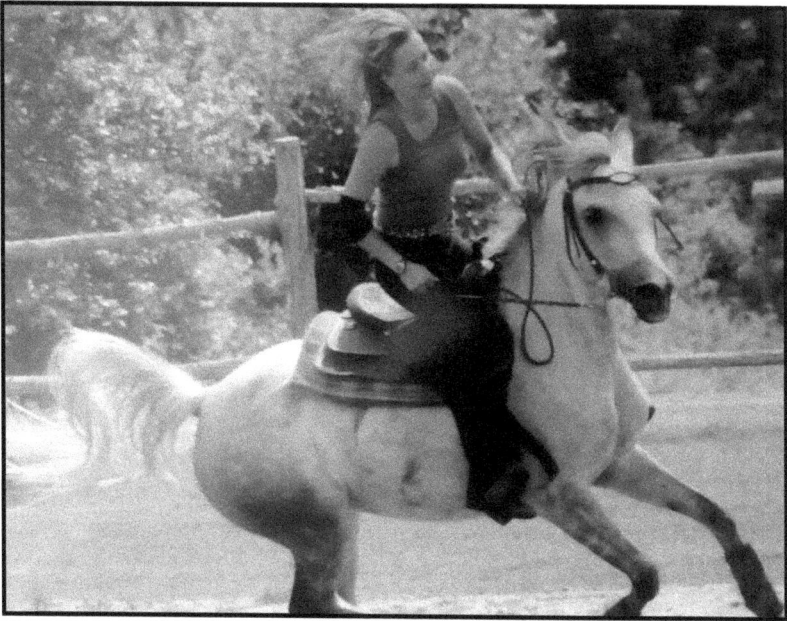

Me (Valerie) riding my Arabian horse, Nicky. Freedom is yours.

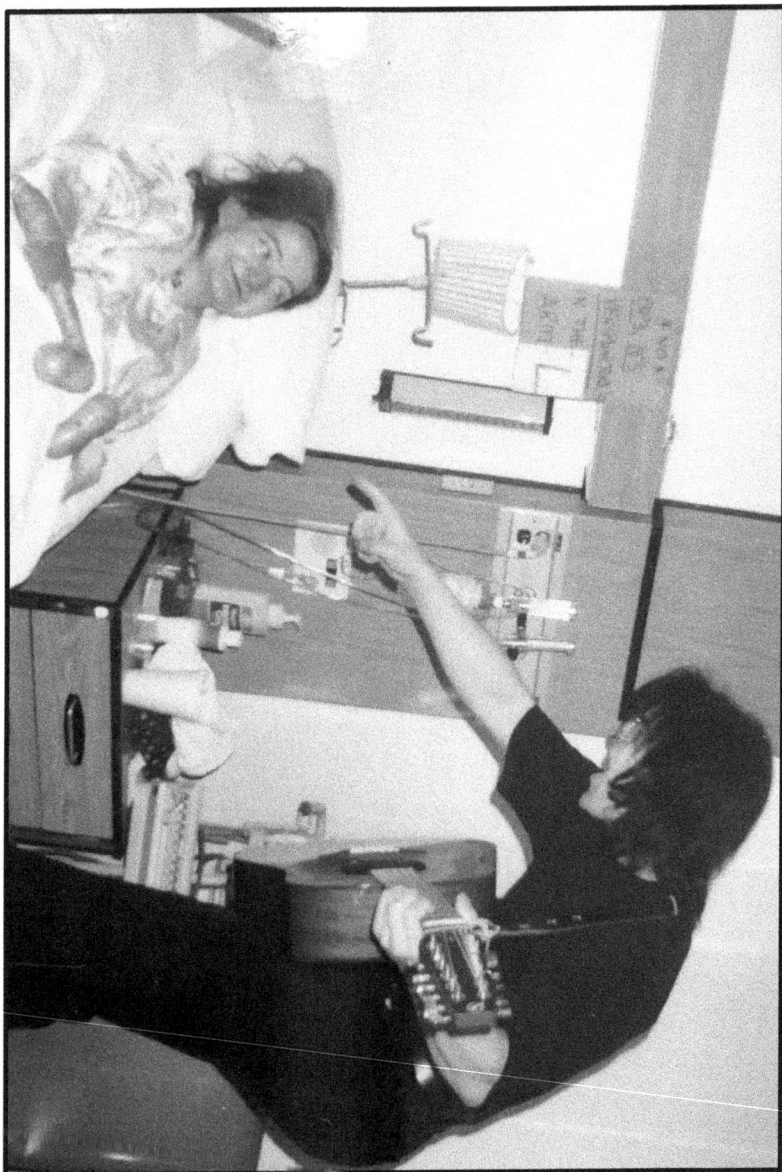

Marlene in hospital with a friend

CHAPTER 9

THE FINAL DAYS

One morning when Marlene woke up, she was coughing, and then she coughed up blood. She was in her apartment in Toronto, at the time. She called 911 and was taken to the hospital. She knew something was terribly wrong. She was told she had a cancerous tumor the size of a grapefruit in her lung. She was really pissed, because she had never smoked a day in her life.

She talked to the doctors to see what her options were. They decided to do radiation and chemo and she went along with it. I remember the first time she was scheduled to do radiation. I had run out to the gift store and bought her a little white stuffed kitten. As a kid, I always would run out and find her a real kitten when she was mad at me.

She thought the stuffed kitten was cute and she decided to name it Radar. She took it into the radiation room with her to keep her company. I still have that stuffed kitten to this day.

For radiation, she was taken into a room and put on a bed that had no side rails on it; plus, it would be lifted up in the air. Marlene was scared of heights and was left in this room alone while she got her radiation treatments. The guy who was doing these procedures was very kind. He told her at any minute he could drop what he was doing and could run into the room to help her if she got scared or hurt.

For her first radiation treatment, I waited outside the room and was pretty stressed out. The next treatment, Marlene was getting chemo. This did make her sick. She said she would have never done chemo or radiation if she had known how horrible it would make her feel. She also had developed a lump on her forehead that was starting to bleed and cause her discomfort.

Soon Marlene would find herself looking at all her belongings and wondering what to do with them all. I remember walking into her apartment and she had all her belongings spread out on a table. She asked me what I would like. She thought I would say her saddle and bridle, but I said I would love one of her horse paintings. She was totally surprised. I picked the painting, and it really touched her heart. She also was a talented artist always painting horses.

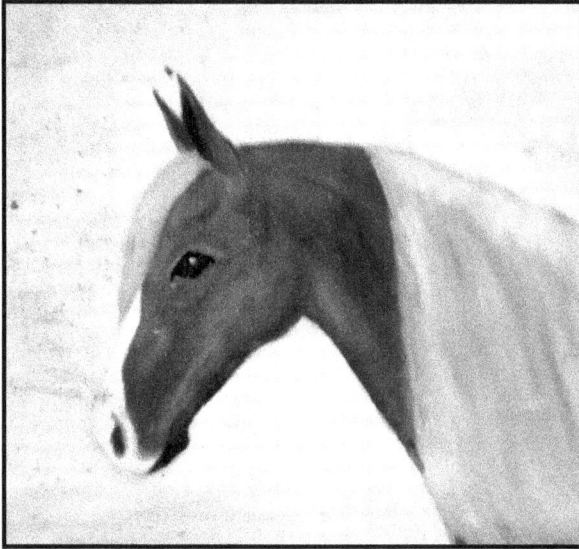

One of Marlene's horse paintings

Marlene was still living in her apartment when she was getting her treatments. My sister, Karen, had come to the rescue. She spent a lot of time helping Marlene. Marlene was grateful Karen was able to come and help her. Karen definitely was a great caregiver to Marlene. Karen also was a good cook and Marlene loved that. Thank God for Karen.

In a short time, Marlene would find herself back in the hospital, and the timing couldn't have been worse. It was 10 days before I was supposed to get married in Saskatchewan. I wasn't sure what to do. Should I cancel the wedding or not? So many people from my husband's side of the family had already bought their plane tickets to fly out for the wedding.

I remember Karen and I having a bit of an argument in front of Marlene in the hospital. Marlene said, "Quit fighting. Promise me you will get along." Karen and I had always had a strained relationship. We weren't very close, but we did get along much better years later.

Marlene then started to go into a coma. We would shake her a bit and she would wake up but then drift back to sleep. She became weaker and unresponsive.

Darlene and Marlene were supposed to go to a concert for a band called Blood Brothers. But with Marlene in the hospital and in a coma, we told Darlene to go to the concert and that Karen and I would stay and be with Marlene. I remember that night very well. It was June 27, 1996. A few more friends had come by to see Marlene. One guy, a musician, came and read her a verse from the Bible. Another musician, a friend named Phil, called to see how Marlene was doing.

The concert was over and Darlene was starting to walk back to the hospital. She had enjoyed the concert. It was music Marlene and herself grew up with. Then at 10:50 pm, Marlene opened her eyes. Her eyes had been closed for days; her eyelids were even stuck to her eyeballs. The day before, her body had become stiff and cold. How she woke up and opened her eyes that night is still a mystery. Karen had yelled out, "Oh my God, she's awake."

Karen quickly grabbed the phone and called our parents. Both my mom and dad were able to talk to Marlene and tell her they loved her. I stood right beside her. I had my hand lightly brushing her left cheek. Her eyes were bright. They even had a bright glow to them. I looked at Marlene and her eyes looked at every person around the room. I will never forget the glow coming from her eyes. Once she looked at every one of us, her eyes fluttered back into her head. It seemed like she was sleeping, when all of a sudden, I said, "Oh my God, when was the last time she took a breath?" We all looked at her chest, waiting for her to breathe again, but she never took another breath.

The room went silent and I quickly ran to the nursing station to tell the nurse Marlene was not breathing. The nurse said she would let the doctor know. It seemed like hours, but finally our doctor came in and confirmed she had passed away.

Darlene was still walking back to the hospital from the concert. I ran out to the door to greet her and tell her that Marlene was gone.

The nurse told us to take all the time we needed to say our goodbyes. We looked around her hospital room and at all her things. I looked at the big roll of cigarette paper and wondered what we would do with that now. There were also her running shoes and her clothes.

Everything was over – all our worrying, all the care we had given all our lives. I remembered walking out of the Toronto hospital at night and a big maple leaf came fluttering down in front of me and hit the ground. I picked up this leaf and still have it in a photo album. I've kept it now for over 29 years.

I knew seeing Marlene wake up after being in a coma for a week that there is more than just this life. There is a white light waiting for us all after we close our eyes and stop breathing. Just like what happened to my dad when he was thrashing, but his journey wasn't over yet and he came back to earth, while Marlene had followed the light to the other side.

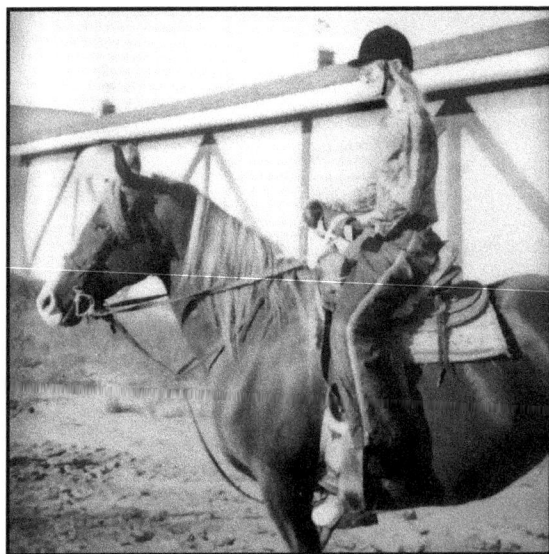

Marlene riding her horse, Basheerah

CHAPTER 10

MY WEDDING

The wedding will go on. My sister passed away on June 27, 1996 and I got married July 6, 1996. On July 1st, we had prayers for my sister's funeral at Saint Julian church. Then Tuesday, July 2nd, we had the funeral for my sister.

Marlene had wanted an open casket. My sister wanted to be seen as she was. She never saw herself as she looked to others. She always felt beautiful, even though her hands were webbed and she had no fingers. She loved her hands because they were different; they were unique. She even wanted her hands to be shown in her casket, but I noticed they had her hands covered up.

Marlene's open casket was located at the front of the church. On the day of her funeral, we, the family, were waiting outside as we were the last to walk in. My mom and dad were out front. We followed them into the church. When my father saw Marlene laying in the casket, he stopped dead in his tracks. We all continued to pile up into each other just like a domino effect. From that day forward, my father started to turn into an old man. He always felt so guilty for bringing Marlene into this world and to live in such pain, day in and day out. Even so, it was harder to lose her. They say a parent should never have to bury a child.

July 3rd, a Wednesday, was the day that separated the wedding from the funeral. Yes, we had one day to mourn and then switch into celebrating. Thursday, July 4th came along, and it was a day to get the wedding rolling.

The guys all went out golfing. They even managed to get my dad on the golf course. The women threw me a bridal shower in the basement of my in-laws condo. We were all just starting to play games and have fun when, all of a sudden, the power went out. My grandmother was a little scared, wondering why the power was out. My fiance's cousin decided to open an exit door which was tucked in behind another building. We all saw dust and debris blowing in. It looked like we were in the Wizard of Oz movie with the tornado.

Meanwhile, all the guys were at a restaurant in Saskatoon. They noticed it was getting very windy. Then, they said the patio furniture started to blow around on the deck. They soon realized it was cast-iron furniture blowing around, so this was no ordinary wind. It was a really bad wind storm brewing.

When the wind storm ended, we made it out of the basement, but the power was still out. My cousin's mini van's driver's window was broken from a shingle flying off the roof.

Another one of my cousins was coming from Alvena to attend my shower when the tornado hit. She was near the Sundown Drive-In when the dust and dirt hit her car so hard that it ending up costing over $5000 in damages.

Ironically, the Sundown Drive-In theatre was playing the movie "Twister" at the time. The sign with the movie name on it had been blown down. I don't think the drive-in ever opened up again after that storm.

The news said it was just a plough wind but if you google it today, the winds were 120 to 140 km/hr that produced an F2 tornado that travelled 13.6 km with a maximum width of 100 metres. The tornado had a track longer than 10 km. The event produced 15 million in property damages. The Texas T, the country bar where my fiancé and I had met, was destroyed. I don't think the Texas T was rebuilt after that either.

Was this a sign that the wedding wasn't supposed to go on? I was starting to question everything after the week I just had. Then, finally, Saturday, July 6, 1996 came and it was a beautiful, peaceful day. As I walked up the stairs to get married, I stopped and looked down at the graveyard and the pile of dirt where my sister was buried four days previously. I thought to myself, "Until we meet again; until we ride again".

Perhaps the wind storm was a message. I don't know, but that marriage didn't survive. Luckily, I later met Mark and we ended up getting married and still are. I ended up having a beautiful wedding without all the drama and without any family funerals overshadowing it. Mark and I have a farm in Ontario where I raise and keep my horses. I am finally living the peaceful ranch life I always wanted.

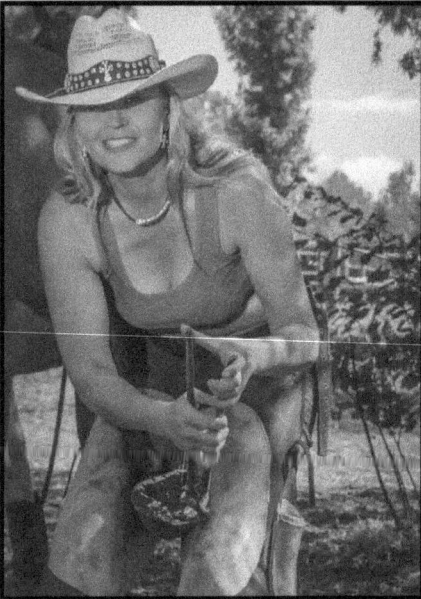

Me (Valerie) working as a farrier – a profession inspired by both Marlene's and my love of horses.

Conclusion

I wrote this book because I really didn't think Marlene's book would ever be published and hers is a story that must be told. My sisters and I each thought we should finish it, but 29 years have gone by and it hasn't happened. So, I have decided to at least get my version out into the world. It is my hope that it will give other families going through difficult times due to a condition or disease of one of their loved one's, peace, hope and the will to keep going.

I hope you have learned from and perhaps been inspired by my account of what it was like to live with someone with a severe case of EB. Even though most of it was very tough (with the toughest part experienced by Marlene), it also provided me with many experiences I wouldn't trade for the world. Marlene really was a go-getter and she reminded me never to settle. Anytime I would think of making excuses for why I couldn't do something, I would just look to Marlene and realize my excuses had no merit.

I will share one last story that I think sums up Marlene's spirit and determination in a nutshell.

Marlene was in Toronto General Hospital. Her kidneys were failing and there were five doctors who weighed in on her case. Our whole family was in the room with her when these five doctors stood around her bedside told her there was nothing they could do for her. They said they could only make her comfortable until she inevitably died. The room went quiet and then my sister spoke. She looked right at the all five doctors and said she wanted dialysis.

The doctors said they didn't know how to give someone in her condition dialysis without harming her further, so there was nothing they could do. She emphatically looked them in the eyes and said, "Who the HELL do you think you are? I WANT DIALYSIS! I AM GETTING DIALYSIS. You're the doctors, so put your heads together and figure out how to do it!"

And by some miracle, those five doctors did. My sister lived on dialysis for over five years. One of the top doctors at the Toronto General Hospital later apologized to her and said she was right to fight for her life, but she shrugged it off.

Marlene was on dialysis twice a week, for 5 years, and it took 4 hours each time. This is when she found the time to write her book.

An example of Marlene's handwriting, which is remarkable given she didn't have fingers. She wrote her entire book by hand.

The doctors also published their breakthrough of giving a person with severe EB dialysis and so Marlene is in a medical journal. She was the first person with EB to receive dialysis in Canada.

Throughout the years, doctors told my parents that Marlene shouldn't have been able to live past the age of five. They had no clue who they were dealing with. Where there's a will, there's a way; and Marlene had more will than any person I have ever known.

Marlene (Oceania) wants to send a message to you. She wants you (and each and every one of us) to grab life by the reins and gallop hard and fast through the open fields, letting nothing stand in your way, because this is YOUR LIFE. Go live it with everything you've got.

www.ingramcontent.com/pod-product-compliance
Lightning Source LLC
Chambersburg PA
CBHW052120030426

42335CB00025B/3070